I'LL NEVER WEAR A BACKLESS DRESS

Sandy Appleyard

PREFACE

I was born and raised in Toronto, Ontario, Canada by my Mother, Father and my older sister Cher. We had a pretty textbook family up until I was around four years old. That was when my parents separated. My mom, sister and I moved out to Malton, Ontario to live closer to my maternal grandparents. My parents separated for many reasons, but mostly because my father had a severe drinking problem. Some family members on my dad's side have said it was arguable whether my dad's drinking became heavy before or after my parent's separation. More of this story is outlined in my first book, "The Message in Dad's Bottle".

I was always sick as a child; whether it was asthma, bronchitis, tonsillitis or ear infections. I was never healthy for my birthday or for Halloween, which are only a week apart. It wasn't until I moved away from my mother in my early twenties that I realized most of my childhood illnesses were likely attributed to the fact that I always lived with a smoker. It seemed like within a month of moving out on my own, all my ailments were cured. To this day, I still remain very healthy, and live a much healthier lifestyle.

One of my passions has always been reading. I enjoyed doing it less as a student, since textbooks are constantly forced upon you. I did pick the hobby back up as a favourite in my early twenties, and now in my thirties I am hooked. The other, rather obvious passion has been writing; since I was a young child. My favourite class in high school was English. I took all my subjects at an advanced level, but my English homework was always completed first.

In elementary school I wrote a story entitled "How The Skunk Got It's Stench". It was a reiteration of a small storyline found in the children's movie "The Labyrinth" starring Jennifer Connelly and David Bowie. In the movie, there is a scene in which all the puppets and Jennifer Connelly are on this trek, in search of her kidnapped baby brother. They encounter many obstacles on their journey, but one in particular was the "Bog of Eternal Stench", which they have to cross. However, their challenge is to cross it from a series of small, slippery rocks covered with moss; and it is said that if you so much as dipped a toe into the bog, you would smell bad forever.

This was my theory, and my explanation for how skunks acquired their unpleasant odour. That story was found to be such a favourite among my classmates that our teacher decided to conduct a lesson in book binding, so we could treasure our compositions forever. I still have that book, and yes, I did treasure it. However, I later learned from my first job as an assistant animal groomer, that my story was incredibly untrue. Animals smell bad for much less romantic reasons!

When reading, I enjoy biographies, historical and current. One of my favourite authors, Philippa Gregory, creates stories relating to real medieval characters. From her, I have read about Napoleon and Josephine, The Boleyn Girls, Queen Katherine of Aragon, and the most interesting in my opinion, was reading about Queen Marie Antoinette.

When reading about Marie Antoinette, I found something about her to be very intriguing. It is such an obscure thing; to find something in common with someone who lived hundreds of years before you. Or rather, something in common with a family member of someone who lived hundreds of years before you. It was Marie Antoinette's son. He was born very deformed, with severe curvatures in his spine. He later died as a small child of lung and intestinal collapse due to complications from his deformities. But he, too, was born with Scoliosis.

Introduction

I have written about a hundred poems during the course of my life, some are featured in my first book. I felt this current book "I'll Never Wear a Backless Dress" was warranted because I needed to express my experiences, both good and bad, in the best way I know how.

In my opinion, Scoliosis has changed my life significantly since the moment I learned I had it. One of the main frustrations in having this deformity has been feeling alone; Scoliosis is not very widespread. My hope in publishing this book is that I can reach out to some who have Scoliosis and feel that same loneliness. At the same time educate their families and friends about the emotional side of the deformity, rather than simply focusing on the physical/medical aspects.

I feel I can reach many audiences; any person who has a physical ailment that affects their daily life can relate to my experiences. You would be surprised how many people in this world suffer from something that causes them pain or discomfort every day. Some issues have either very little or no treatment available. The same is true for Scoliosis.

I had heard, while doing some of my own personal research in the past, long before starting this book, that there was a procedure some elementary schools performed in the past, in order to detect Scoliosis in children. With the student standing bent over, the school nurse would place a device similar to a ruler or level on the child's back horizontally; perpendicular to the spine. This procedure would be repeated in increments down the length of their back. If the straight edge was unbalanced at any point, this would indicate the possibility of Scoliosis, and prompt further medical testing.

Of course, this method was unscientific, and required further testing and/or x-rays to properly diagnose and determine the extent of Scoliosis. But at least it helped in early detection. Early detection and treatment is best, since most curves can be corrected and possibly reversed while the child is still growing. Most treatment is performed by one or all of the following methods: exercise program to stretch and strengthen the curvatures appropriately, bracing to stabilize and/or offload and correct (similar to orthodontic braces), and finally the most extreme: surgery to realign the spine via rods, screws and/or hooks placed along the curve(s).

Unfortunately, none of the schools I attended performed any such procedures. I wasn't diagnosed until my early twenties, by which time it was far too late.

Chapter One

I remember in elementary school; when all the children sat in a circle on the library floor while the teacher read a story, I was the only kid who couldn't sit up straight. All the other kids had their legs crossed over Indian style, and they were sitting right up like a bunch of little soldiers. As much as I tried, I could never do it. I was always slumped over, or I had to lean on one arm for support.

Throughout my teenage years, I always felt there was something a little off about my body. I noticed I would always have pain in my left shoulder blade. My Mom always thought it was premenstrual. I also noticed in all pictures taken of me during my teens, my right shoulder was always higher than my left. Shirts never seemed to fit correctly; they would always fall to one side. Necklaces would always sit unevenly on my chest, and the clasp would always fall down until the pendant caught it. Bra straps always fell down on one side, purses never stayed on my shoulder. I always wore my purse like a messenger bag to compensate. My ponytails, if worn at the base of my neck, would always inch to the left.

Even during high school and college I noticed my backpack was always drooping to one side. Of course, any back problems would have been exacerbated by the amount of textbooks I always had to carry around throughout high school and college. The worst was across college campus, I had a fifteen minute walk to class from my car on any given day. I estimate that my accounting book alone had to weigh at least ten pounds.

I had a little pot belly that I could never lose, no matter how many sit ups I did. When I was researching pregnancy once my husband and I started to try for a baby, I read somewhere that if the paternal genes are in any way altered, the fetus can be deformed. For example, if the father consumes drugs or alcohol while sperm is being manufactured, the genetic information can be damaged, thus causing birth defects or disfigurement. I don't have any proof of this. However, my father was an alcoholic long before I was born. There is only one family member who has Scoliosis, one of my aunts on my mother's side. Although hers is very mild and she only has one curve.

It's difficult to say whether I have more of my mom or dad's physical features. I have always had large feet (size ten-actually they have shrunk for some reason in the last few years to a nine). Although I am only five feet three inches tall. My mom's stature is much like my own, short and average build. My dad was tall at six feet even, and very slender. My sister is tall and, up until having my niece, was also slender. My dad always told me my big feet would pay off because I would be tall. I stopped growing basically around the time of his death when I was sixteen. Although, if you consider how much length I probably have lost in my spinal curves, that could probably account for some lost height.

I remember when I was about twenty three; I was sitting on the floor in the recreation room we had in the apartment where I lived with my mom and step dad. My mom came in for a minute to watch some television with me; I got up on my knees to switch the channel, and my Mom noticed for the first time that I had a hump on my back. Neither of us thought anything of it at that time. She just thought it was the way I was reaching over to change the channel.

It wasn't until I experienced my first car accident about a year later that Scoliosis was discovered. I originally went to physiotherapy to be treated for whiplash after the accident, but upon my assessment, the therapist took one look at my back and told me I had Scoliosis. I had no idea what that meant, and I just said sarcastically "well, that's just great". She ran her finger down my spine to illustrate the curves, but it still never occurred to me just how bad this was, or how much this would affect my life.

After treating me for the whiplash and some soft tissue injuries, they began casually treating me for the Scoliosis. They began with some light exercises and stretching to add to my own personal workout that I had been doing at home. About nine months after that accident, I unfortunately was involved in another car accident (please note that both these accidents were investigated by police and were not my fault). Fortunately, this accident wasn't nearly as bad (my car was written off in the previous one), but was way more terrifying (I was sandwiched between two transport trucks on a busy highway-neither of them saw me). So, I was once again placed in physiotherapy for whiplash.

At this time, my boyfriend and I moved into a rental apartment together about a half hour away from where I was currently living. Thus, I had to stop attending that physiotherapy clinic. I thought I would be alright without it for a while, so I didn't seek out a new clinic. This was fine for a couple of months; until I suddenly started to experience constant nauseating headaches. This prompted a doctor's visit; and he gave me a requisition for physiotherapy. The new clinic initially treated me again for my neck injuries directly related to the headaches. But once that was over, they started to treat the Scoliosis with essentially the same plan as the previous clinic.

Chapter Two

My job at the time was as an administrative assistant for a large, growing company. When I say growing company, I mean GROWING. We had such high turnover with employees that some would leave during the first day because they couldn't keep up with the demand. One of my coworkers had a tradition whenever another employee would leave. He would play the song "Another One Bites The Dust" by Queen at his desk, where a lot of people would congregate. We had a laugh, and he was great. My daily tasks involved a lot of desk work; including phone, emails, data input, and filing. My responsibilities there were anything from Accounts Payable and Receivable to working with customs for clearance of our trucks to sales invoices…you name it, I did it. I loved it; I was great at it, and I absolutely loved everyone I worked with. I worked there for five years and loved every minute of it.

I had all the amenities within the office that I needed, including a headset to assist with answering the phone, an ergonomic office chair, I even had a step stool to prop up my feet to alleviate some back strain. All of these things were simply not enough to ward off back problems. The physiotherapist who was treating me at the time urged me to get up at least every half hour and move around, and she gave me a series of stretches to do during my lunch hour and breaks. Unfortunately the job, with the sheer volume of tasks alone, did not enable me such breaks or even lunches for that matter. This fact came crashing down on me when I started having back spasms. That first one I had was a real eye opener. All I did was get up from my chair to go use the washroom. The minute I got up I felt like something was gnawing at my lower back. Every move, no matter how little, was very painful. I couldn't bend to sit back down, so I had to grab hold of the filing cabinet to stabilize myself. The only thing I could do was flag down a coworker to have them assist me. I was finally able, after a few minutes of no movement, to inch myself back into the chair. This whole incident took about half an hour. Once I sat down, I called the physiotherapy clinic. They were able to see my right away. I have no idea how I drove there, but I remember when I got there, I walked slower than a snail to the door and luckily someone saw me coming, so they opened the door for me. I had to get the receptionist to remove my shoes for me. That was probably my most embarrassing moment. I lost three days from work, and attended four or five physiotherapy sessions in between. I didn't feel normal until about a week later. I had ruptured a disc in the lumbar region of my spine.

Chapter Three

Shortly after my first back spasm, my boyfriend and I bought a house in a town about fifteen minutes away from our apartment. I immediately looked for a doctor in the area, and was fortunate enough to find one about our age, and right up the street from us. My former doctor, even though I was in his care since birth, was located at least a half hour away from where I lived throughout my life. Plus, since my new doctor was young, he was very in tune with new medical breakthroughs, procedures, etc. So it was definitely a win win situation for me.

I guess with all the right things happening in our lives at the time, I figured everything was good, including my back, so I foolishly did not look for a physiotherapy clinic again. The headaches returned. Then my back started to be bothersome again. Instead of simply giving me a requisition for physiotherapy treatment, my doctor decided to send me for some x-rays, and refer me to an orthopedic surgeon.

It was about a six month wait to get an appointment with this particular surgeon. On the day of my appointment, as I was driving to the office, I noticed it was in a rundown area. The office was full of papers and older style equipment. If someone lit a match, the place would be up in flames before you could blink. The waiting room was about the size of a local area mall washroom, and there were about thirty people crammed into it. There were no windows and not enough chairs to seat everybody. I had to wait about three hours. Now, think about this situation: a room full of people with physical ailments, some who might not have a chance to sit down for an unknown amount of time. Not to mention, these places require you to bring your own x-rays to your appointment. I personally had to carry this sandwich board sized paper bag containing my x-rays, which I knew I had to be careful not to bend or rip it in any way. Do you think these doctors think of these things? I doubt it.

I was called up to the reception area to submit my x-rays, so the doctor could review them prior to my appointment time (which, by this time was about two and a half hours ago). Then I was asked to complete a customary document so they would have something to line my file with before the doctor made notes of his findings. Are you familiar with this document? It is a badly photocopied sheet of paper with check boxes and obscure questions like dates and situations that nobody could possibly remember unless you personally carried your own medical files along with you for every appointment. I take this clipboard (shocking, they actually supply you with a clipboard....and a pen....that works), and try to find a chair so I can complete it. At least I am now minus my sandwich board sized x-ray bag, so I might be able to complete it.

Have you ever tried to write on a clipboard while it is upright? It is virtually impossible, plus, the pen stops working because gravity sucks the ink back too far for it to reach the tip. So you are left to bend forward, holding the clipboard in your lap…but wait……I have Scoliosis, do you think after sitting for practically three hours that I can bend, especially after having to get up once and sit back down again? It makes me laugh to think of the insensitivities that exist in the medical world. The one thing that they want you to do you can't, and that's why you're there to see them. They would never have thought of that. I thought it was the medical secretary's job to know what a person's medical issues are and what they mean. That is why we need a requisition from our doctor in order to get these specialist appointments, right?

That's not all. I manage to complete my form somehow, and then I finally get called in to see the doctor. I probably should have told you that I never looked at my x-ray before this appointment. All I did was get the x-ray done, which is nothing unusual except that the x-ray is taken while you are standing. The doctor welcomed me into his office and did the usual "how are you today?" crap and wrote a few notes down. At this time, he asked me if I had been to physiotherapy and I said yes, then he asked me to bend down and touch my toes….wait…BEND DOWN….TOUCH MY TOES?????…..did this guy know anything about Scoliosis??? I obliged unwillingly. I managed to bend just a little less than forty five degrees or so. And that's it. He did nothing more but state that if physiotherapy is working then I should continue my life normally and see you, have a nice day. Bye. He handed me back my x-rays and sent me off on my way. Keep in mind I still have never seen my x-rays. He left the office and I began to put on my jacket, and I thought to myself: I am curious; I should look at these x-rays. I opened up the bag and pulled out this life size x-ray and nearly fainted.

My back is shaped like an "S", and not a small, vague little one, we're talking a fifty five degree angle going one way, and a forty seven degree angle going the other way. Continue my life as normal????? Are you insane?????? Oh my God, this is *not* normal. This doesn't even *look* like a back; it looks like some kind of evil serpent of Hell or something. How am I supposed to live my life? Have a family? What will happen when I get older? What are the complications I can expect? About a million questions were going through my mind as I'm sitting there crying, all alone. I can't leave without asking him some of these questions. It's not right; he didn't even ask me if I had any questions, he didn't even show me my x-ray. He knew I didn't open it because the seal wasn't broken. Did he ever even think that maybe I might not know a lot about this? I thought that was his job: to explain it to me?

I managed to compose myself and clean up my face a little. I got up and headed over to the reception desk. On my way there, the doctor sees me again. I asked him the simplest question: can I have a family? He answered 'oh yes; don't let anyone tell you because your back is curved that you cannot have kids and you can't live a normal life'. He said I should consider myself lucky that my curves are almost equal in their angle, so they almost offset each other completely. Thanks.....consider myself *lucky*? What kind of a person says that to you? I am aware that I don't have cancer or some other nasty disease, so yes, I am lucky for that, but I should think I'm lucky for this? To top it off, years later I obtain my medical records from my doctor; and lo and behold, I see this doctor's notes. He says in his notes that I will be looking at reconstructive surgery in the next five years or so....did he even mention this to me???? NOOOO!

I guess it was my own naivety and therefore my own fault, for not researching Scoliosis once I was diagnosed. I was young....live and learn. I could use all kinds of clichés to rationalize why I didn't do my homework. I should have gone into that appointment with a list of questions and concerns, especially since I waited so long to see the doctor. When we are just starting out in adult life, I think we carry on the ideal in our minds that doctors will make us better. When we are children, we go to the doctor with mommy or daddy, he or she gives us medicine and all is well. Take two of these and call me in the morning, you know? I thought it would be that simple; surgery or it will go away itself or something like that. I kick myself now for being so stupid in thinking that the x-rays were the hospital's and doctor's property, so therefore I wasn't allowed to open them or look at them. You would think at age twenty four I would know better; not so much. Once again, having Scoliosis has opened up my eyes, and I've learned a lot about it and so much more.

Chapter Four

After a little while, I took the doctor's comments with a grain of salt. I found myself a wonderful physiotherapy clinic less than ten minutes from my house, and they were open evenings, so it was perfect. The bulk of my treatment to date has been acquired from that clinic. They have been wonderful to me since my first day; very accommodating and understanding, and most importantly, very caring.

I went through a little turnover in the beginning because not only was I new, but they also had a few new therapists. It was funny because part of their protocol was to ask you how you were feeling when you first arrive. For the first little while, as I was still getting accustomed to the clinic, I though they were just being polite. So I would answer, Pretty good, how about you?" Dianne didn't say anything for about a month, and then she started being more specific, "how is your neck, how about your back?" Once I realized, especially after hearing the other therapists ask the same question to their clients and listening to their responses, I felt like such an idiot!

Thankfully that was one thing I loved about Dianne, she had a great sense of humour,and she was very patient. After getting to know me and my body, she only asked that to actually be polite, because this woman was like a physical psychic. She knew just by watching me walk in and get up onto the bed, what kind of shape I was in. She could even tell which joints were stiff, how much of a headache I had, and when she succeeded in relieving my headache. When my back was in spasm or just stiff and sore, she knew what treatments I would be able to handle, which ones were out of the question; and most of all, she knew when she did a particular treatment on me, that I might have some issues getting up, so she always assisted me.

The best thing she did for me was create a vigorous exercise and stretching program. She would book me extra time with her about once a month to review them all, and watched as I did them and made adjustments where applicable. She would give me the simplest ways to know if I was doing them right or wrong so I wouldn't injure myself, and how to advance them so I could challenge myself without getting injured. Best of all, she took the time to write them out and give simple illustrations so I could remember how to do them until I got used to them. She had the best descriptions for the exercises, too, like the "happy hooker stretch". She would even ask me during the month if any were getting too easy for me, just to check and make sure I was doing my homework. She always made sure I was pain free and had no stiffness before I left the clinic, and kept working on me until that goal was reached.

That to me is what a physiotherapist should be. She was so supportive, even throughout my pregnancy, when things got really challenging for her. She still worked on me without reluctance. Once I was seeing her for about six months or so, she even put me on a program where I was given a discounted rate since she knew I would be what she called a "lifer". She knew I would always need to come to physiotherapy; that I would never see my discharge papers like most of the clients at the clinic. We also had this understanding that if I felt like I needed a break from the clinic and from attending physiotherapy (which I never did), that I could just call at anytime to come if I needed to, and she would fit me in. Dianne was amazing at what she did and for good reason, not only was she incredibly smart and very well accredited, she had also been doing it for something like twenty years. So, unfortunately, she retired from the profession about three years after I started seeing her at the clinic. Sigh.

Chapter Five

Rob and I bought a house together. It was the perfect location since it was exactly thirty five minutes to both our places of employment. It was fair in distance for each of us to travel to get to work. Rob's job entailed a lot of driving to offsite locations, but he was still required to go to "the shop" every morning, and then be sent off to the job; wherever required. My job, however, was stationary, and it was pretty simple to get to. The long drives in a low riding vehicle weren't doing my back or my neck any favours, so we decided to buy a sport utility vehicle instead of my current sedan. This vehicle was just my size; it was dubbed "the cute ute". It was small enough that we didn't need running boards for me to enter it, but it was tall enough that I could open the tailgate and get my groceries or cargo in without having to bend at all. The driver's seat was just perfect for me, and the blind spots were so minimal.

My back and neck were behaving well now; I had a great physiotherapist, great new car, Rob and I were well on our way with making wedding plans. I was doing well with my daily exercising, stretching and strengthening. One question still remained in my mind...could I have kids? It's not that I was questioning my ability to conceive, it was more whether or not I could carry them during pregnancy. What would I do about having an epidural? Once Rob and I were married, we immediately started trying for a family. There had been some issues within my immediate family with conception and delivery anyhow; so I thought there was no time like the present to start a family.

Getting pregnant was a slight issue; it took eight months. I think it was more so because of my stressful job than heredity, because once I had my first child, I stayed home with her, and then getting pregnant the second time took only a month. Once I was pregnant with my first child, in my opinion, it was a tough pregnancy. Overall, I got huge. I gained just thirty three pounds, but I was really big in the baby area. I had Braxton Hicks (false labour) contractions from twenty four weeks (six months) until the end. I have to say though, I was extremely lucky with my back. To my surprise, I suffered no back spasms, just a lot of pain and frequent tightness. I kept up with my exercise program right up until the day before I delivered her. Exercising made me feel great, the time I spent exercising was the best I felt during the pregnancy. I also saw Dianne right up until the week before I had Olivia.

The terrifying part was the labour and delivery. Olivia came seventeen days early, although that wasn't a surprise to me because I was incredibly large and very ready. My water broke on queue-in bed in the middle of the night, and the labour started immediately following. The unexpected part was that my contractions started and continued at two minutes apart, and it was all active (painful) labour. So, I was terrified because while doing our birthing plan, I thought I would try to avoid an epidural, but at this point it was inevitable. I didn't even want to think about it, I had heard so many horror stories about the possibility of becoming paralyzed after an epidural, or having chronic back pain indefinitely. That part didn't bother me because I had that already, but could it be worse pain? More often?

What's worse is that when the anesthesiologist came into the labour and delivery room with the medication, he seemed very inexperienced and unsure. He told me that I should have had a consultation with him beforehand......HOW SHOULD I KNOW THAT???? SORRY, you want to have one NOW??? So I bent over the bed like he instructed me, and held Rob's hand. When the doctor was finished inserting the needle into my back, he said in a very hesitant tone "well, I think that might work".....suddenly, Rob fainted. Poor Rob, he later commented that he couldn't believe a doctor would say that or behave that way. He feared the worst; that I would be paralyzed and he would be left to look after this new baby by himself and his wife for the rest of their lives.

Fortunately, everything was a success. Olivia was born in perfect health, I was fine, and Rob regained consciousness. Motherhood was a challenge, unlike any other I had ever experienced. Olivia was a wonderful baby……during the day. She didn't sleep through the night until she was eight months old. She was also an incredibly large baby; ironic because now we can't keep the weight on her. I decided to breast feed her for many reasons, but above all, because it was the best for her. I enjoyed having large breasts, too. If the size of your breasts is supposed to be directly in proportion to the size of your baby, that would explain a lot.

Breastfeeding was very rewarding, but it was also very challenging for me physically. Dianne had to work extra hard to keep my upper back happy because of breastfeeding posture. My neck suffered a little, too, because you have to look down a lot to ensure the baby is feeding properly and not snoozing on the job. Thus, my physiotherapy visits were growing in number; which was difficult to juggle with a new baby. After having Olivia, we decided we weren't going to have any more children: we had our hands full and were quite happy with just one child.

When Olivia was about four months old, I went back to my doctor to ask if there was anything else that could be done to help me. The physiotherapy/babysitting juggling act was growing very tiresome on Rob and I, and the medical bills didn't exactly fit our budget under one income. Rob's medical insurance only covered my physiotherapy expenses for approximately half the year. My doctor asked if I would like to go back and see the orthopedic surgeon. I flatly declined. His solution was to visit a different surgeon in a different city. He also gave me a requisition to have a pulmonary function test. The purpose of this test was to see if my curvatures had affected my rib cage to the extent that pulmonary function was compromised. The test consisted of checking breathing and heart rate, as well as lung capacity.

That test reflected no issues thankfully. The next orthopedic surgeon wasn't as horrible an experience, but it definitely did not make me much happier. For this one, it was a party of three. Since Olivia was still really small, both Rob and Olivia had to accompany me. Which I thought would be a great idea. The waiting room was small, but it was okay because there were only two other families waiting. We were escorted into the doctor's office after about a twenty minute wait, so that was definitely good considering Olivia was with us. Once we were in though, it was a different story.

The doctor once again had a preliminary review of my x-ray prior to my appointment time. Instead of having me bend over and possibly inflict pain, he had me stand in front of him and explained the location and severity of my curvatures. Once I sat down, he started completely out of left field…..talking about cars with Rob. Comparing Volkswagons to others and such like that. For about ten minutes the two of them went on and on. Then he moved on to Olivia. He started playing with her. I have no issues with any of this….AFTER we've discussed why I'M here. So I intervened. I started asking my battery of questions. He stopped me after question two-is surgery an option for me. He said exactly what the other surgeon said, that if physiotherapy was working for me, than I should maintain that. He also said that if I were a candidate for surgery, he would be happy to recommend one to me, but that he wouldn't feel comfortable performing the surgery himself. OK…YOU are an orthopedic surgeon. Apparently he should be an auto mechanic, because he seemed to know more about cars. If he didn't feel comfortable talking to me about my back, than he should have referred me to someone he felt would feel comfortable. Now, in retrospect, I understand that I might not be a candidate for surgery, but his job was to explain why. He gave my husband and daughter more time, WAY more time than he gave me. I left there feeling cheated and alone. At least this time I didn't feel stupid, like I did with the last surgeon.

I was so frustrated, not only with both surgeons, but now with my husband, for not encouraging this doctor to address the issue at hand. I thought considering that we were now in this together with a child, that he would be on my side. Somehow I felt he wasn't.

If that is one thing I have felt having Scoliosis, it's that nobody else understands. Nobody is willing to help me except my physiotherapist, who sees me every week and knows the pain and discomfort I feel. The only other person who is truly sensitive to my experience is my mom. She is the only one who makes me feel like I'm heard. When my back hurts, she offers to carry stuff when we're shopping together, she helps me up and down when I have to sit and I am showing a little pain in my face. Nobody else does that. When she comes over for a visit and we don't have enough seating, she sits on the floor and lets me sit on the chair while her husband and my husband sit on the couch and play with the PlayStation 3. She gives me the best seat in the house when we go over to her place: her chair.

My mom is also the one who praises me when she hears that I still haul my ass out of bed at 5:15 every morning, so I can do my exercises before my kids wake up. Even when I only had three hours of sleep for ten and a half months when my second child had colic; she was the one who praised me and kept me going when I could have cried I was so tired, but I knew if I didn't exercise I wouldn't be able to look after my children. My mom would also come over and help me bathe Olivia when I was pregnant with my second child, because my back was so sore and once again, I was so large with my second pregnancy.

One of my other frustrations is that some people think that because I am at home with my children that my life is easy. I know the old cliché that staying home with your children is the most difficult job in the world. Yes, some days it is for most stay at home moms. That's why most would rather go to work and earn a living to pay for daycare expenses than stay at home with their kids. It's been a huge sacrifice; leaving the job I love, living with no extra income and sometimes just having enough money to buy food and nothing else. But top that off with getting up as stated above, at 5:15 in order to be on the exercise bike by 5:45 and finished all my exercises, strengthening and stretching by the time my baby wakes up. I pray to God every night that my back is alright each and every day, so I can look after my kids. I cross my fingers during each morning workout that my back doesn't go into spasm, or get injured before I'm finished. Not to mention, trying to get through each day looking after the girls and doing housework without doing any damage to myself. I also have to ensure that my kids' schedules coincide with my physiotherapy schedule.

Chapter Six

Once Dianne retired, of course they had to place me with someone else. Michelle was new, and I was new to her but obviously not to the clinic. She was much younger than Dianne and even younger than me. I chose her because the clinic was going to place me with the owner, but her schedule was mostly days and I needed someone who I could see during the evenings. So, Michelle it was. At first, I wasn't sure if she would be able to meet my needs because she was so new. But it didn't take me long to realize that she was indeed very able.

Michelle immediately did some review of my current exercises and printed off some new ones for me to try. She had some new methods as well, which had been quite successful. I still maintained my relationship with my massage therapist, and she concurred that Michelle was great. Michelle updated her education regularly(as if she didn't have enough credentials); this girl meant business. She was serious about being as good a physiotherapist as she could be.

Rob and I had originally decided after having Olivia, that we would not have another child, but after seeing families with one child and the obstacles that they had to overcome, we made a decision to try for a month for another baby. My guess was since it took eight months to get pregnant with Olivia, I had a slim chance of getting pregnant that quickly. As fate would have it, I became pregnant in that month.

Shortly after I started seeing Michelle was when I became pregnant with my second child. I could tell this made Michelle excited, but at the same time a little nervous about treating me. This pregnancy was much different than my first. I was so sick with nausea I had to be put on Diclectin for the first six months. Starting in month five, I had Braxton Hicks contractions. I had back issues, hip issues and foot issues. As if that wasn't enough, in my last two months I suffered from sciatic nerve pain; which meant I could only sleep lying down and I could only lie down if I had an ice pack on either side of my groin. I had to walk around all day long with an ice pack on my back. Sleeping was almost impossible because if I were to lie on my side for more than ten minutes, my hip would ache on that side, so I would have to flip over. I haven't been able to lie on my back in years because of the Scoliosis, so being pregnant and lying on my back was not possible. I managed to maintain my weight and still exercised every day up until the day before Victoria was born, as hard as that was.

I was glad Victoria came early; in fact, she was nine days early. But again, I was so huge that I knew the baby would be born early once again and sure enough, she was. My water broke again in the night while I was in bed. This time though, I was so relieved the pregnancy was going to be over; I was so relaxed. I didn't even wake Rob up until 6am, well after calling my Mom at 5am to tell her not to go to work, that it was Baby Day. I was so calm; I barely even felt the contractions start. I took a shower at my usual time, although I did skip out on exercising that morning, just to be safe. I wanted to *walk* over to the hospital so they could triage me at 10:30am; that's how calm I was. My mother almost fainted when I told her that, she insisted Rob drive me over with her.

When I got to the hospital, I was already six centimetres dilated, but my contractions were bearable. I sent Rob to go buy a new toaster oven with Olivia, and then told him to take her home for a nap. Little did I know my labour was progressing very quickly. So quickly in fact, that Rob missed the delivery. The nurses barely got my shorts and shoes off in time for Victoria to come out. Thus, no epidural was administered.

Chapter Seven

After having Victoria, all my back issues were returning, plus new ones, so Michelle thought it was time to consider other possible alternatives. There is one great advantage to having a new physiotherapist, and that is, for the same reason I love my family doctor: they are aware of new professions, procedures, equipment, etc. So, Michelle introduced me to the idea (after having shared with her my previous two experiences with orthopedic surgeons) of going to see a physiatrist. The physiatrist, as it was explained to me, functions as the go to person for the entire medical field, when all other treatments/medications, etc. have been tried and failed. This medical profession is relatively new, and therefore Michelle thought it would be a great idea for me to consider trying.

With physiatry being a relatively new profession, and the way the current medical system is run, the waiting lists are endless. Michelle knew of one particular physiatrist from a contact at the University she attended. She helped me set up an appointment through my doctor's referral (she even wrote a letter personally to my doctor), and walked me through what to expect, what I should think about asking, etc. My family doctor even tried to set me up with their physiatrist, just so I could get in with someone, either one, as quickly as possible. The wait for the one Michelle set me up with was about seven months.

While waiting for my appointment day to arrive, I had to have another back x-ray. Fortunately, it reflected no real change in my curvatures. So, having Liza didn't really affect my back negatively thankfully. Rob took a couple days off so he and the girls could come with me (again, it was necessary because Liza was so small). This time, the appointment was in a hospital. I remember the day was probably the most windy it had ever been in my memory. We went for lunch just before the appointment so both the girls would be fed and happy, since the appointment was just before lunchtime.

When I arrived, after filling out yet another file liner, I noticed there was a disclaimer on the question sheet. It said that if the physiatrist offers you any medication, that it is your right to ask for it in it's generic form; and that you are not obligated to purchase anything. Red flags kind of went up for me, but I didn't really take it to heart since it didn't affect me.

I was brought into a room, and the way it appeared to me, I expected to see a bunch of beds within a ward. I think they turned the ward into a medical office, but kept one room for the patients being examined. So I sat in this room, two doors away from Rob and the girls, alone. I could only hear people whispering because they probably knew if their tones were any higher, that I could hear them.

I sat and waited for about forty five minutes, after the first girl who brought me in asked me to remove all my clothes except my underwear and socks, and gave me a hospital gown. So again, I have Scoliosis, and they have asked me to sit on a hospital bed in a cold room with a hard floor. Alone, behind a curtain…for forty five minutes, while they do God knows what. Suddenly, this guy came in and introduced himself. I knew he was not the physiatrist. He looked at my sheet (which he'd already had for a while, plus my x-rays), and started asking me some simple questions. Then he asked me to verify the name of the physiotherapy clinic that I attended, since I'd only written its name in the short form (I didn't think it mattered), and he asked me how long I'd been at physiotherapy. He explained that he was an orthotist; and that he was a person who fitted people with orthotics for shoes, braces, and things of that nature. He said he didn't feel that he would be able to help me, since I was already fully grown, and that back braces were generally helpful only to kids and teens. I knew that, but thanks anyway.

Thanks....bye. The doctor will be by shortly to see you, he said. Five minutes passed, no doctor, but Mr.Orthotist returned and asked me if I'd yet tried physiotherapy.......Okay, maybe *you* need therapy more than me, I thought to myself. Then, as if I thought this couldn't get any worse, he came back in and asked me to twist to the right. I was ready to clock him. People with Scoliosis (with two curves) generally can't twist to any degree; I knew I couldn't unless Michelle forced me over and then did some stretching and mobilization so I could twist a little for a couple days after my treatment (improving my range). I looked at him, and I think he realized how senseless his request was; so he actually used his brain and told me how to do it in such a way that I could. Wow, so you aren't completely useless, I thought. He gave me these subtle little movements with my shoulder, ribs and torso, so I could twist. He asked if it was painful. I felt like asking him which part......him or this movement he was making me do?....instead I was nice and I answered no.

He recommended that I be fitted for a brace that would help force me into this position so I could twist on my own. Then, he went into this whole sales pitch about the newest, latest and greatest model of the brace. This brace, by the way, he told me is worth $3500.00CDN, and was probably not covered by health insurance. By this time, I had completely lost interest in him and in this whole physiatrist thing, and was ready to leave. Then he left and said he would return with a prescription for the brace.....oh joy.

Just then, the actual physiatrist came in with another little friend. One who was probably no more than eighteen years old, I'm guessing. She didn't ask me if I was okay with having an audience present, but told me the girl's name and that she would be joining us. Great, so now I'm a freak. She had probably never seen anything like this, so she was rounding up a student as a witness…..."Hey, you'll never believe what I saw today…..no no, ask her, SHE was there with me!!!"…..seen in Physiatrist's World Today magazine. I'll bet.

The physiatrist did not really examine me, except for having me turn around and face the wall, while she showed her little friend my curves, and how my shoulder blades were uneven as well as my hips. She did measure my leg length; to try to rule out the possibility that maybe the cause was that in fact my legs were uneven. They weren't uneven any more than average. She did ask me how much relief I got from physiotherapy, but she didn't have many questions for me; or any answers.

I had no trouble with the physiatrist's bedside manner, she was perfectly polite, and I believe she gave me as honest an opinion as possible. But I was truly disappointed because she offered me nothing. She concurred with all others in that physiotherapy was the best treatment for me. She said the only way surgery would be an option for me, is if I began to have neurological problems, or issues with pulmonary function. Even at that, if I was cured surgically, I would be opened up and sewn up from the bottom of my neck to the top of my buttocks, and I would have absolutely no range of motion at all. Essentially my back would be fused together via rods and screws and I would only be capable of up and down movement. There was also no guarantee that I would live pain free. The surgery was too risky, and therefore the issue was not discussed further.

What was discussed further was the idea of this brace. Moments later, Mr.Orthotist returns, and then they both decide to tag team me with the idea. They were like used car salespeople: "this is the greatest thing on Earth, you won't even be able to tell you're wearing it", "it's made with the best fabric, and you get three pairs of shorts with it", I know a dancer who uses it", and the best was " it is so new that we haven't even used it on children, since we don't have any data available on it's long term effects, we are currently only using it on adults"....great; so now not only am I a freak, but I'm also about to become a guinea pig.

I stopped them when they explained the cost of this thing, and said that there was no way that I could afford it if it wasn't covered by medical insurance-as they claimed it usually wasn't. This is where I lost all faith in humanity. The physiatrist turned to me and said that they could work out a payment plan, or sometimes they were willing to have you work at the manufacturing lab in lieu of the costs. I was thinking to myself, for starters, if this thing is so new and isn't even being used on the general population, why is it not free??? Second of all, you want a person with severe back problems to work? At a manufacturing lab, no less? Not to mention, I have already informed them that I am a stay at home mom with two kids to look after: do you think I can work? Do you think that is an option for me?

I left there crying. Nobody was really truly willing to help me. In my opinion, these people I have seen were just in it for the money, or just doing their job. In situations like this, you need someone who is willing to go above and beyond for you, and I guess those people just don't exist in the medical world today. I did get honesty; I'll give them that, which is more than I can say for the first two doctor's visits I had. But nowhere did anyone come out and say 'hey, this lifestyle is not working for you, here's what I can do to help'.

Physiotherapy is not a long term plan, at least not a successful one. Michelle was at her wits end with me because she couldn't help me more. She worked on me once a week and I still only got a day or two, maybe three, of some level of pain relief. What happens in ten or twenty years? What about supplementary issues like arthritis? I did a lot of research, and there is a list of about thirty things that are common for Scoliosis sufferers in the long term. Not to mention, I looked in to this brace when I got home from the physiatrist appointment. Sure, the website for the brace said, and showed actual illustrations of people who did get somewhat better after using the brace. But they neglected to tell you what can happen in other cases. There is some offloading that occurs initially when you start using the brace, essentially removing stress off some parts of your body that are experiencing pain, which in turn relives some of it if not all for some length of time. But, what they don't tell you is that the possibility of your back actually getting worse if you stop using the brace is quite high. Some Scoliosis sufferers had minor curvatures upon initially being fitted with a brace, and then afterwards, their curves were so bad that they actually needed surgery. What happens is that your muscles that are normally used to support you in those areas (and would be toned and strengthened to do so) where the brace removes stress, they become weak and thus when the brace is removed, your back can no longer withstand the stress again, causing your muscles to give and thus creating a worse degree in the curves.

I decided, despite the bleak outlook on the brace, that I would submit it to our insurance company, just for kicks. Although, I was pretty sure it would be a letdown, since our insurance company made no efforts to keep us happy over the preceeding year. They lost a couple of claims, which I had to hunt down not once, but twice. Then, Rob had to fight tooth and nail for at least six months to have them cover his sleep apnea machine. So, needless to say, my hopes were grim.

Chapter Eight

During the time that I was pregnant with Victoria, Michelle and I started discussing the possibility of me returning to work. This, of course, would come after Victoria was at least a year old. Originally, when Olivia was born, Rob and I decided that I would stay home for several reasons. It was mostly a financial decision at the time. But, it was also because deep down I knew that I couldn't go back to a desk job. Time and time again, while I was seeing Dianne, she told me that a desk job was torture for my back and neck.

Each time I sat down for more than about twenty minutes, I would effectively squish the discs in my vertebrae. The discs were under risk of being ruptured each time I rose from a seated position for that length of time. The same held true for my neck, although I didn't suffer from neck spasms, rather severe headaches (sometimes even migraines). When Olivia was about two years old, Rob and I decided I should try working again. But, instead of a desk job I tried something retail.

The job I accepted was at a local card store. I figured it was perfect; light work, no computers, and it was part time. My first shift started out fine; they did some training on how to use the cash register, how to organize and place the cards properly in the display, and generally where to look for things, etc.

For the first half hour I was okay. Then, my feet started getting sore, and then my lower back started at about an hour into the shift. They tried to show me a few things in the back, as far as closing procedures, and I knew I was in trouble. I bent down to see what was done at the register, and I could feel my back screaming at me. When I got home, I knew the second I sat down, I wasn't getting back up. I sat down, and I ended up sending Rob out to the drugstore to get me some muscle relaxers and my ice pack. I had to sit for an hour with the ice, and I waited until the medication started to work, before I could make my way up the stairs to attempt to go to bed.

After this, Rob and I were scared. What kind of work could I do? Desk work was out of the question, the same for retail. What kind of job exists that does not involve sitting or standing for an extended length of time? The only job that I can do is being a mom. My job at home allows me to do things at my own pace, and I can stand up or sit down as often as I need to. Plus, if my back or neck bothers me, I can look after it from home.

We decided that we needed to look into the possibility of applying for disability for me. The first thing that I did was discuss this with Michelle. She told me just to look it up on the internet to see what was involved. She thought I would definitely be a good candidate for it; that the career choices for me, in her opinion, would be very bleak. I was shocked because before mentioning disability to her, I figured she would look at me like I was being totally unreasonable. In my mind she had probably seen truck loads of clients with Scoliosis and other debilitating back deformities. Her response was although approximately half of her clients had some sort of Scoliosis; I was her worst case.

That fact terrified me. Michelle looked at me differently from that day on. I think she really connected with me, especially while we were going through the application process. She even told me she would contact Dianne and have her complete a form for me as well, given that Dianne did do the bulk of the treatment up until that point. The support I received from them, and from my family doctor, was wonderful.

The application process was very long and enduring. It took over two months to get all the information together, have all parties involved complete their portions, and have almost everything sent together in one complete package. It was grueling. My own portion included about twenty pieces of paper; dates, times and explanations of things from over ten years ago at that point. But I was thorough, as were all the others involved. I even included a letter explaining the time line and purpose for each clinic I visited, and all other important items that could not be listed on the application.

I admit I was a little concerned. I feared that the appropriate people would not be reviewing my case; I doubted a physiotherapist would ever see my application forms. Both Michelle and Dianne's portions contained a lot of medical information that only someone who was familiar with musculoskeletal issues would understand. Dianne and Michelle stated very clearly that I was very compliant with my home exercise program, and that I regularly attended physiotherapy, with the same physical complaints. This, according to Dianne, holds more water than someone who periodically comes into physiotherapy, and complains one visit of one ailment, and the next visit complains of another. Which held true in my case; I would come in each week with a headache due to neck tension, very stiff back and rib cage, and as of late, since having Victoria, I would have pain in my rib cage.

I also found, along with my medical file supplied by my family doctor, that the physiotherapy clinic had submitted periodic reports to my doctor, updating him on the progress of my treatment. It was very consistent, and it coincided with my information and my knowledge of what my current physical situation was in the last six years since I had been seeing the doctor and attending the clinic.

The only documents that concerned me were some that were submitted by the two orthopedic surgeons. They supplied my doctor with more information than they supplied me with. For example, I wasn't told by the first surgeon that I may require reconstructive surgery in the next five years or so. And the second surgeon said that he would recommend having x-rays and a follow up appointment with him every five years. Things like that disturbed me, and made me glad, if nothing else, that I went through this whole process and uncovered all these facts that I would otherwise have never known about.

The application forms stated that it could take up to six months for the review to be completed, so I didn't expect to hear anything until the summer time, when I had only sent the forms in just after the New Year. Suddenly, in early March I received a letter stating that I had been denied. At first, I couldn't believe it, I was so disappointed. Rob's first response was that I wasn't quite broken enough, so I still had to work in the government's eyes. I repeatedly read through the explanation, and gave up. Personally, I thought that if I fought further, that they may try to prove that I was somehow embellishing the truth, and therefore they would defame me. I wouldn't let someone make me feel like I was trying to fake anything. That wasn't me.

After giving it some more thought, I decided that if I stood by and just accepted it, that they would be proving that I believe I don't actually qualify for disability. And that I was just testing the waters to see if I could get it. Rob also believed that maybe the initial denial letter was a method to weed out the ones who are trying to ride the system, and that I should refute it.

I took a couple days to digest the honest truth about how they did review my case and decided that they didn't give me a fair review. The first thing that stood out was how fast they reviewed my case. I sent them a very large manila envelope, at least an inch in thickness. They took the time to list all the documents they addressed in their review; which totaled four. The actual amount of separate documents I sent them totaled twelve.The other important factor that sent red flags up for me was the person who signed the denial letter. The person was signed 'RN', which of course means 'Registered Nurse'. I consulted Michelle, and she confirmed that there was very little chance that a nurse would be qualified to review any type of musculoskeletal issues. I thought about the possibility that this nurse was perhaps just the person who completed the administrative portion. This did not make sense to me; if they had a doctor review my case and had an administrative person complete the denial letter, they would have either signed it "per", or the doctor would have signed it, and the administrator's initials would have been after the salutation.

Another issue was that they did not have anybody interview or examine me. There wasn't any proof that they viewed my x-rays, and they therefore did not see the x-ray reports. Further, they tried to deny that I qualified to apply for disability, since I had not worked in the three years before applying. They neglected to acknowledge that I was home caring for my children, there was a form for that too, that they missed. That part really irked me because if you aren't able to work, you wouldn't be, would you? But in order to qualify for the benefits, you must have been working in at least the last three or four years (they gave the time in weeks) prior to applying for benefits.....interesting catch twenty two they put you in.

Lastly, they said that because I didn't take pain medication, and have adapted my lifestyle to accommodate for my physical needs, that I wouldn't qualify for benefits. This was infuriating. I don't take pain medication because I cannot. I had an ulcer in my teens, as a result of stress when my Dad was ill with alcoholism. The only pain medication that I can take is an over the counter muscle relaxant, which I cannot take while I'm caring for my children because it contains codeine. Codeine is also an addictive and/or habit inducing drug that I will not take unless it is absolutely necessary.

My pain is controlled solely by physiotherapy and daily exercise. Any pain that I suffer in between must be accepted and dealt with as best as I can. I have to understand my limitations, and so do my family and friends. My house is relatively clean, but cleaning is done in bits and pieces. Our house is in terrible need of work, but most of it has to wait, since we have only one income, and I cannot work-even part time.

So I took all the above retorts, and sent in an Appeal Letter. I also listed the documents they did not acknowledge, and resent them with my letter. I argued with them on several other smaller issues, but the most important points were mentioned above. My appeal letter was sent out exactly a week after receiving my denial letter.

In the interim, this was at the same time when I would be receiving my appointment with the physiatrist. About a month and a half later was when I received the call from Service Canada. The lady had originally left a message on our answering machine, saying that she would call me the following day at a specific time, so I was to expect her call. I thought this was a little strange, and wondered why she hadn't left me a number so I could return her call.

When she called the next morning, she asked me a couple of questions, just to reiterate some of the simple, but important points in both my application and in my appeal letter. Then, she said that based on the information that she had contained in my file that I did not qualify for disability. Apparently, since I did not take pain medication, and I seem to be able to care for myself, my home and my children, that I would undoubtedly be able to handle the demands of a job. I maintained my composure to a point, as I realized this woman would probably be the last person to review my case, and I didn't want to be foolish and insult her, for this might change her decision if she did have any chance of approving me.

I was strong in my conviction that I have tried a desk job and a retail job and have failed at both. I also explained my reasons for not taking pain medication. Finally, I stated to her that in my opinion, I did not believe that there was a job available that would enable me to sit down or stand up as much as I needed in order to avoid pain. She responded by saying that it was not her job to find me employment. A few other words were exchanged, and then she said she would be in touch with the physiatrist for her opinion if I would be physically capable of working. After that, I knew I would be denied again.

After several follow up calls I finally received a final denial letter, approximately three months later. The physiatrist apparently did not have any evidence that I was unable to work based on her knowledge of me during my short appointment with her. They offered me a chance to present my case to a tribunal. I declined. I had to because it would require a lawyer to submit my case and support me, which we couldn't afford.

Chapter Nine

After a few months of liaising back and forth with our benefits supplier, surprisingly, I was given approval for the back brace. I had several consultations with the orthotist before receiving it of course, but once I had it, for a few months, I thought it was the greatest thing since sliced bread.

If you observe me wearing it, it definitely resembles something out of a bad S & M movie. All I would need is a whip and some chains, and I'd be all set. He sent me home with a diagram outlining how to wear it, and the correct application process; which was very important since if it was worn improperly, it could cause more harm than good.

The whole theory behind it is to literally force my body to correct its posture, and in doing so relieve pain. It is also intended to help with support, since my whole carriage (rib cage) area is generally weak. Historically speaking, since I learned I had Scoliosis, my pain free standing time was limited to about twenty to thirty minutes, depending on what I was doing. After having the brace, and using it regularly for about a week or so, I was able to double my pain free standing time. This meant I had more freedom to do more things I had not been able to do like baking, and generally standing around (!)

The down side to the brace was that it was terribly uncomfortable and hot. There was no way to wear it during warmer months, especially considering you have to wear it over the supplied body suit, or a pair of shorts and t-shirt. Driving with it on was extremely uncomfortable, as was wearing it while sitting for any length of time. Also, it took forever to remove and replace when toileting. The most critical disadvantage to it was that after using it for a couple months, my neck started to suffer. My guess is that because it forced my shoulder blades to straighten, that caused my neck to be offline. I had to unfortunately stop wearing it because of inconsolable neck pain. Yes, it was in fact, a pain in the neck!

Chapter Ten

While writing this book, I had been home with my children
for four and a half years. I did make an honest attempt at a
home based part time job. It was a Telemarketing Company,
its headquarters were in Saskatchewan. While it was a
wonderful company with great people to work with and for, I
could only do it for about three months.

My letter of resignation stated that my reason for leaving
was to accommodate for my husband's working hours during
his peak season. Given that I had to work four nights a week,
starting immediately at 6pm, Rob had trouble making it home
by that time and he was forced to turn down overtime work.
Truthfully, I left because I just couldn't stand another minute
of it. When I first started, I loved it. They had me on a
particular project that I enjoyed and was doing well at. Then
suddenly, during the Christmas holidays, my supervisor
telephoned me and suggested I join a training session for a
new project upcoming in the New Year. I was given no
information about it except that I would make substantially
more money. I was also given no time to think it over or to
discuss it with Rob. So of course when a carrot is swinging in
front of your face, you grab it right?

Wrong. They kept telling me I was doing great, even though I wasn't getting any sales at all. Then, finally when I was starting to get sales, I only got them for a week, then not again. I asked to be put back on my original project and they declined. After a month of this, I had enough. They tried to persuade me to stay, but I wasn't having it. The good thing is that they said should I want to return at anytime, to give them a call. At least that was an option. The only reason I could physically handle that job was because I was doing it from home. I also received a headset as a gift, so I was hands free. It was a little constraining though, because I had to put my phone system on standby periodically throughout the night so I could stretch, since the system would automatically display client information simultaneously as you received calls. So I couldn't just walk away from my desk, I had to be looking at it since the call would come in and you had to know who to ask for that second.

During the time that I had taken that job, it quickly occurred to me that I had to change up my physiotherapy schedule. I had been attending therapy on Thursday evenings, and once I started the job, I had to work that evening. Schedules conflicted, resulting in me having to go to therapy Friday mornings…..which meant I had to bring the kids with me…..ohhhhhhh the fun!

I began seeing one of the owners of the clinic. I had seen her briefly before, and I started thinking that maybe this was for the best. The reason I say this is because I felt that maybe there was some frustration in the clinic surrounding me. I got the feeling that maybe they didn't know what to do with me anymore. In that industry, they are typically used to clients coming in for a prescribed amount of time based on their physical needs, and then they are discharged. In my case, that would never happen. Sometimes I felt like I should change clinics, just for some new blood, but then I was reluctant to do this because they were so good to me.

Once the children began to feel comfortable at the clinic, they of course, began to misbehave closer and closer to our arrival time. This made it very awkward for my therapist to treat me, especially during massages because I was so tense. Also, my therapists spent more time babysitting some days than looking after my physical needs, simply because of my body positions, since I couldn't see the kids myself.

So I was kindly offered another option. There was a new therapist, just starting out at the clinic. She worked Monday and Thursday evenings, so back to evenings I went. The only difference was my appointment time. I chose to have my appointments after the kids had gone to bed. This offered me so much more freedom. I was able to prepare the kids for bed and put them to bed as usual, and then I would proceed to the clinic…alone.

The best part of this was that I was the last client for my therapist on Thursday nights, so I had her all to myself. This meant she was focused only on me and my time spent there was minimized. I was typically at physiotherapy for about an hour and a half to two hours previously, now my time there was reduced to only an hour, sometimes even less. This was great. Karen was great, too. She was my age, with two small children herself, so she and I could relate to each other's challenges in life. Also, she was very capable of treating my condition and often did quick techniques on the spot to cure my pain.

My most recent annual physical revealed that I have not shrunk again, contrary to my thoughts. My doctor also discouraged me from getting another x-ray since I only had one a year ago. Apparently the Scoliosis series x-ray is very high in radiation exposure, since you must have your entire trunk (skull to pelvis) x-rayed. Therefore, he explained that I should not have them repeated unless required or requested by another doctor. Which lead me to my next question for him that day; I have noticed that I do require pain medication more often now, mostly for my neck, and I wondered if he might consider referring me to yet another orthopaedic surgeon. He once again discouraged this since in his opinion, another surgeon would probably have disappointing news for me as well. Plus, I am currently still on a waiting list to visit another physiatrist (this physiatrist evidently takes a few years to get in to see).

Chapter Eleven

A friend of mine started talking about the wonders of yoga about a year ago. She attended the new "Hot Yoga" variety. I put it in the back of my mind at the time, but then just recently another friend who suffers from back pain also marveled on the wonders of "Hot Yoga". So I asked her if she would recommend it to me. She stated that since she started it about four months prior, she has had zero pain relapses. So, yes, she highly recommended it to me.

So I looked into it of course. The "Hot Yoga" classes, while they sounded absolutely wonderful and right up my alley, were a little inconvenient and didn't fit our single income budget. So I thought to myself, well heck, I've been doing my own exercises at home for nearly fifteen years, why should this be any different? So I went to Wal-Mart and bought a Yoga DVD.

I must tell you, anyone who has any kind of back or neck issue should definitely try yoga. While mine isn't "Hot Yoga", in my opinion, it works just as well as long as you're completely awake and warmed up. I have found a little pain if I do it too early in the morning, and my body isn't quite up to it yet. But if I do it a few hours after waking up, it does wonders for my body.

I started doing it about five weeks ago, and I have told everyone who has asked me, that it has changed my life. My neck and back have never felt better. It is ingenious the way they have set it up. You must work your way up to different levels so you won't hurt yourself. Also, if there is a pose that I can't do because of my back (and there are a few, trust me), I substitute in exercises from my regular routine instead. It works out great. I do this twice a week, giving myself at least a day or two for a break, and in those days I do my regular exercise routine (which is a half hour on the exercise bike, followed by about the same amount of time for floor exercises supplied by my physiotherapy clinic).

Since adhering to this new exercise schedule, I find that my body feels so much better. I am not waking up in the night with my neck hurting nearly as much, and I haven't once awakened with a sore neck in the morning since I started doing yoga. I have more flexibility in my lower back, and more strength overall in my whole core section.

I think when you have back or neck issues, you are reluctant to try something new, for fear you are going to hurt yourself. In my opinion, I think most people who suffer from pain, use it as an excuse (whether consciously or not) to steer themselves away from doing exercises. I'm obviously not trained in any medical profession, but I think that we all need to try things within reason, and find something that works. The more you sit and do nothing except rely on pain medication, the less progress you will make.

Even if you try physiotherapy, they will recommend exercises to do in order to help rehabilitate yourself. But if you don't attend regular physiotherapy, you must try something to get yourself active again. The more you sit and gain weight incrementally (which will happen the less active you are) the worse your pain will get. It will become a vicious cycle and eventually you will be immobile. This is a fact that I have been told by my own physiotherapist. I cannot gain weight or my entire back will no longer be able to support my body. It was a sheer act of God that I was able to carry both my children to term.

Chapter Twelve

Once I started researching Scoliosis, I encountered some information on a few famous people who have it. There is a world renowned golfer and a pool champion who are among them. What I thought to be a little too cliché was that they stated they never let Scoliosis get in the way of their dreams. Whenever I hear this, whatever the case, it always gets my attention. There are some people in the world who truly cannot achieve their dreams.

Mine as a teenager was to become a veterinarian. When I was in high school, I worked myself sick to maintain my grades because I was trying to get into the only University that offered the Veterinary Medicine program in the province I lived. I could not handle the pressures of maintaining a high ninety average in my grades in order to be accepted into that program. Not only did I have school work to deal with, but I was also dealing with a very difficult life at home. My father was suffering terribly with alcoholism, and he later passed away when I was sixteen. I still graduated from high school with Honours, but my grades were inadequate for the program I dreamed of.

As an adult, my dream is to become a registered dietician. I have always been a person to lead a healthy lifestyle. I started exercising in my early twenties using an exercise video that my mom and I purchased, and then I moved on to the exercise bike. I have continued to exercise every weekday since then. I have never smoked in my life, never really drank, and I have always maintained a healthy weight. I have always wanted to help others achieve the same healthy lifestyle. I have also been very fascinated by the workings of the human body. If I ever had the stomach for it, I would have loved to have become a doctor. But truthfully, I believe my calling is to become a dietician.

I have researched the program at the University of Guelph, where the program is offered which is close to where I live. It is a four year program. I physically cannot do this because it requires sitting in classrooms for four plus years of my life. It is longer if I want to be a registered dietician. This makes me feel like somewhat of a failure in some ways.

This, however, is completely untrue. If it were true, I would probably have become a person with very low self worth, and I would have invited everyone to join me in my pity party. I would likely not exercise at all, having given up hope; thus, I would be overweight and in very poor health. Plus, if I was overweight, I would likely be completely disabled and/or bedridden/wheelchair ridden. It would be very likely that I would have also taken up alcoholism, since that is in my family. I would probably have never gotten married, nor had any children.

I truly believe that one day I will be able to become all that I want to be. There are online classes that have become available in the last few years, and although they are expensive, it is something that I can start with one day. Perhaps even one day we will all be able to complete programs and degrees like this online. So I haven't given up hope of my dream.

I did accomplish one dream last year by publishing my first book "The Message in Dad's Bottle". So, things can happen when you put your mind to it. It took me three years to write that book, and although it was done in bits and pieces over time, I completed it. So you see; it doesn't matter what challenges life throws at us, I truly believe that God never gives us more than we can handle.

When I think about whether or not I want to feel sorry for myself for having this condition, I consider other people who are way worse off than me. You see people every day who are plagued with serious physical illnesses or challenges. And I believe that my life could be much worse. Given the severity of my curvatures, I am blessed to have the amount of physical freedom that I do. And I realize that one day I might not have that. Just like everyone else in this world. You can have an unfortunate accident, or become ill any day of your life. We all take risks every day; when we drive or fly or even walk across the street. I take as much care of my body as I can every moment as a result.

Chapter Thirteen

I simply cannot complete this book without telling you about
my husband. We met when I was twenty four and Rob was
twenty five. I had just moved out on my own for the first
time, having just acquired my first job outside of graduating
from college. Rob was living with a friend of his at the time.
We actually met online. I did not find good sense in meeting
men through the bar scene given my family history with
alcoholism. I was also working for a company that consisted
mostly of middle aged men. So, online dating was my best
course of action, since I did not want to be alone.

When we met, I had just been involved in my first car
accident. I still have the very first emails we ever exchanged.
When I look through them every so often, I realize just how
lucky I am. The emails I sent to Rob were so self involved and
full of self pity. I felt so sorry for myself for being in an
accident. Ultimately I was fine, but I kept harping on how my
arms hurt and how I had this ache and that pain. I was
surprised he held in there.

He fell in love with me fast and hard, and I wasn't quite
ready yet. He was patient with me. When I found out I had
Scoliosis, he wasn't scared off. He should have been. I guess
in all fairness he probably didn't realize how this would
impact my life or his. He supported me in my decision to stay
home with Olivia. He knew that he would be responsible for
the financial support in our house from then on.

He still kept going despite all the stresses of his job and within our marriage. What is truly remarkable is that Rob wanted to be with me. Despite my minor disfigurement and the fact that there were so many other risks involved with Scoliosis. He still loved me no matter what. He knows that I may never be able to work again, and as much as I want to try working again, he always tries to sway me against it. Many people in my life have told me that he is probably just too comfortable because he comes home to a happy, healthy and clean home each night. But I know that is only a small part of it. He wants to see me grow old with him and enjoy our life together, and he knows that if I return to work, that might not be possible.

Chapter Fourteen

The rough draft of this book was completed just before my first book was published in September, 2010. I spent two years sending this manuscript out to publishers and agents to no avail. In that time I wrote two other books and began one other. After two years of shelving this book I looked at it again. It is utterly amazing how different my life and writing style has changed during this time.

Because of finances and my husband's job relocation we moved from Milton to Niagara Falls, Ontario. Life is good here. We can afford things that we never could before and if I can't ever work again it's okay as long as we stay here. My dream has changed dramatically. When I first wrote this book I wanted to be a dietician. My ideals changed while coming up with other ideas and options for myself given my financial and physical situation. It was funny because while I was trying to ultimately figure out what I wanted to do when both my kids were in school full time, I was writing. Isn't odd how what you were looking for was right under your nose the whole time?

In terms of my physical being and how I've progressed in the last two years, I can honestly say I'm doing great. I still go to physiotherapy weekly and I love my new physiotherapist and clinic. It took some getting used to like everything else, but they are very good to me and I'm just as lucky as I was before I moved. I cannot stress enough how much my exercise program has changed me. All I can say is: Yoga. Saved. My. Life. I've been doing it for eighteen months and it has been nothing short of a miracle. I do that along with some lower body strength training and pilates for my abdominal muscles, but *yoga* changed my life.

I chose the title for this book for the irony of it. The irony is this: I did wear a backless dress. It was my wedding dress. I did not choose it solely because it was backless, but because it was beautiful. And when it comes down to it, it doesn't really matter if you try to hide your imperfections or not, it is you that the world will see. People who love you won't care if they can see your imperfections, because that's who you are. Imperfect and beautiful.

Please enjoy the cover of this book (if you purchased the book prior to 2015, or if you have the print version). That is my favourite picture of all time, and it is hung in a large 14" x 14" portrait in our living room, for everyone to see. It doesn't matter if my back is curved, or if my husband's collar in uneven, or my dress is a little crumpled, or my shoulders are uneven. You will never hear me say "I'll never.....anything". But you will especially never hear me say "I'll never wear a backless dress".

The End

What did you think of the memoir? Please leave a review.

No Thanks, Mommy, I Peed Yesterday

Victoria lifted up my shirt and poked my belly button. Olivia shouted, "Don't, Victoria, someone might be in there!"

Olivia screamed from the bathroom, "Mommy, my leg came out!" So I ran, freaking out....it turns out her pant leg was inside out.

Do you have kids? Do you sometimes want to send them to their bedroom until puberty? And other times, do you want to hug them until they burst?

What about those moments when they say something so innocent and incredibly cute or hilarious that you wish you had a pen and paper so you could remember it?

Well, that's exactly what I did. My children have given my husband and I so many gifts, but the most precious has been laughter. I made a record of each funny or cute thing that they said since the moment they could speak.

It's all here in this short yet unforgettable 'Kids Say The Darndest Things' style memoir.

No thanks, Mommy, I peed yesterday is a witty, side-splittingly funny comedy that can be enjoyed by both young and old.

The humorous comments, explanations, and kid-thoughts will stay with you for years to come!

The Message in Dad's Bottle

My father was an alcoholic all his adult life, and the disease took his life at the age of forty-one. When I was ten years old, I became exposed to alcoholism. This book describes what I saw, my reactions to it, and how each situation made me feel. Most importantly, this book illustrates how these factors shaped who I am today. It also focuses on the experiences of others in my life and how each coped with their own alcoholic family member. Included in this section is helpful advice from each person to those who may also be touched by alcoholism. I also share with the reader some of my poems that I have written to help me deal with my past and explain the significance of each.

Other Books

To Hide in Holly Springs
Blessed and Betrayed
Betrayal Only Comes in Green
Seven Lies, Four Truths
She Only Speaks to Butterflies
When Will Knocks at Your Door
Would You Still Love Me?
The Man with the Black Belt
The Message in Dad's Bottle
I'll Never Wear a Backless Dress
No Thanks, Mommy, I Peed Yesterday
Misunderstood
Decisions
Complicated
The Wife of a Lesser Man
Don't Mess with Daddy's Girl
The Wheels of Change
A Coupling Conspiracy
Twenty One Days for Liza

Author's Note

Thanks so much for reading I'll Never Wear a Backless Dress. This memoir was written at a turning point in my life. When I was torn between feeling remorse and anger, coming to terms with a few painful realities, to learning that life really isn't as bad as it seems and things happen for a reason. I wrote this book in less than three months…a big difference from taking two years to write my first memoir. The words and emotions just flowed onto the pages!

Want to know when I have a new release? Sign up for new release updates by visiting my website www.sandyappleyard.com.

Thanks so much for your support!

~Sandy

www.ingramcontent.com/pod-product-compliance
Lightning Source LLC
Chambersburg PA
CBHW060002300526
45794CB00003B/1056

* 9 7 8 1 4 7 5 2 3 6 5 9 0 *